THE CHEAT SHEET

To Get the Pelvic Floor Back in Action

2nd Edition

A Short, Introductory Guide to Gaining
Control of the Bladder $ Pelvic Floor

Joanna Bilancieri, DPT
Author, Illustrator

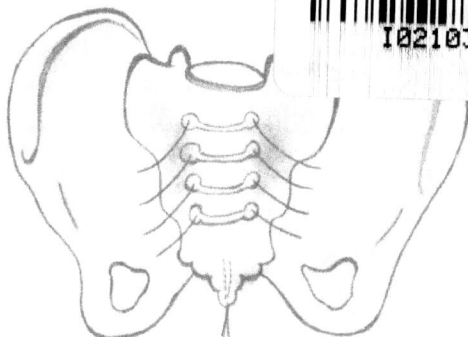

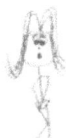

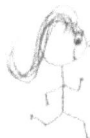

I0210363

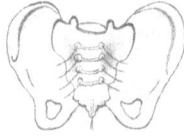

Haven't Got Time for the Full Read?

Based on my publication, 'Get the Pelvic Floor Back in Action', the 'Cheat Sheet' aims to provide a quick reference to pelvic floor exercises and relaxation techniques that can assist in overcoming leakage, urinary urgency and the need to frequently fly to the restroom, and pelvic floor muscle pain. The intent of my full text version is to share my clinical findings and gathered opinions that may be of benefit to those with pelvic dysfunction. If you want to read about the specifics of diagnoses and success stories, please refer to my full text version. If you already know the details of your condition and want to jump into exercises that can assist with pelvic floor control, then jump in here…

Table of Contents

Intro   2

Common Causes for the Need to Squeeze!   5
    Stress Urinary Incontinence (SUI)   6
    Urinary Urgency & Frequency   8

Now Let's Get the Pelvic Floor Back in Action!   9

The Almighty Kegel!   10
    Contracting the Pelvic Floor Muscles   10

Pelvic Floor Exercises   14
    Kegels   14
    Sustained Kegels   14
    Quick Kegels   15
    Timing   15

Combatting Urinary Urgency & Urinary Frequency   17
    Suppressing an Unwanted Urge to Urinate   18
    Timed Voiding   19

Pelvic Floor Muscle Pain & Incomplete Voiding   20

Releasing Pelvic Floor Muscle Tension   21

Helping the Bladder to Fully Empty   22

A Few Words Specifically for Men   23

Outro   25

References   26

Notes/Logbook   27

Disclaimer

The author, illustrator, editor, printer, formatter, and publisher of this book recommend seeking medical attention for medical advice. The contents of this book do not substitute for the medical attention and/or the needs addressed by individuals' clinicians. The author, illustrator, editor, formatter, printer, and publisher of this book intend to present correct information at the time of press. Any and all information utilized is at the reader's own risk. If any techniques, exercises, treatments, instructions, and/or other materials are utilized, the reader does so at his or her own will and risk. Any performance or use of the techniques, exercises, treatments, instructions, and/or other materials is at the reader's own will and risk and should not be performed or utilized if any harm or pain develops or worsens. The author, illustrator, editor, printer, formatter, and publisher of this book do not assume and do disclaim liability for any errors and/or damages resulting from any cause.

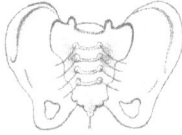

Common Causes for the Need to Squeeze!

Conditioning the pelvic floor muscles with exercises called 'Kegels' can help overcome many conditions. Common calls to strengthen the pelvic floor stem from urinary leakage with activities such as running, lifting, sneezing, coughing, and laughing, and the need to run to the restroom as soon as an urge strikes. Other conditions involving urinary system malfunction and pain can benefit from training the pelvic floor muscles to release their tension. As stated in a later section, this release in muscle tension can help one to fully urinate and can help to reduce pelvic floor muscle pain. Releasing excess pelvic floor muscle tension is oftentimes easier after a "squeeze", or Kegel. Therefore, Kegels are important when trying to strengthen pelvic floor muscles *and* when attempting to release their tension. The sections below briefly describe common conditions beckoning a Kegel, and a later section will share some of the conditions benefitting from a Kegel followed by a concentrated release.

Stress Urinary Incontinence (SUI)

Stress urinary incontinence (SUI) is aptly named because when physical *stress* on the pelvic floor overwhelms pelvic floor muscles' contractile abilities, it can lead to involuntary urinary leakage. Sneezing, coughing, laughing, changing position, catching a ball, running, or otherwise jolting the torso can increase pressure and apply a force on the bladder. Such a force can simulate contraction of the bladder's detrusor muscle, whereby the urine presses forcefully against the internal sphincter and the external sphincter. With greater pressure applied to the pelvic floor muscles, their constituent fibers have to work harder to hold the external sphincter closed.

Ha Choo!

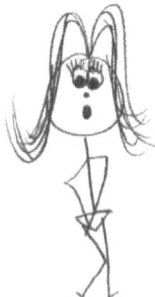

Here is a comparison of the bladder without (top) and with (bottom) extra intra-abdominal pressure.

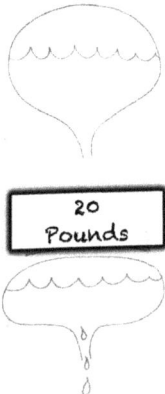

With pressure applied to the bladder, as with coughing or sneezing, urine can seep through the sphincters beneath the bladder. On the left, an *inadequate* pelvic floor muscle contraction (a weak or non-existent Kegel) leads to incontinence. On the right, an *adequate* pelvic floor muscle contraction (a strong Kegel) counters the pressure applied to the bladder and prevents unwanted urination.

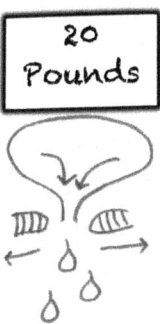

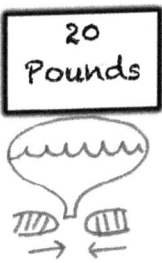

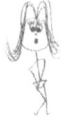

Urinary Urgency & Frequency

Urinary urgency and frequency are characterized by the *need* to use the restroom before the bladder is full, otherwise leaking occurs. We are normally alerted to seek a restroom when our bladders are partially filled. With a partially full bladder, we can normally walk calmly to the restroom to void. When a partially full bladder suddenly strikes up an urge and results in an all out sprint to the restroom, there is a problem. When urine leaks in conjunction with the sudden urge, especially without having a full bladder, there is an even bigger problem! Frequency follows urgency's lead to the restroom, characterizing the *need* to urinate *more often* than when the bladder is full.

Urinary urgency can lead to frequent trips to the restroom, otherwise leakage can occur.

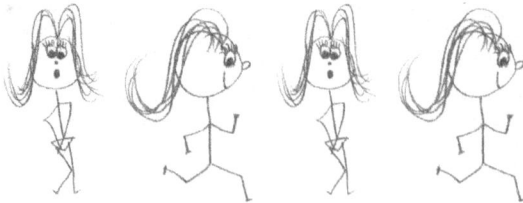

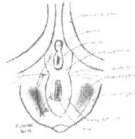

Now Let's Get the Pelvic Floor Back in Action!

Below are explanations of how to exercise the pelvic floor muscles, or 'Kegel', and how to time the Kegels to effectively overcome conditions requiring control of the pelvic floor. The exercises aim to strengthen the pelvic floor muscles by increasing their force of contraction, length of contraction, and agility needed for implementation into daily activities.

Kegeling correctly can take some time! Persevere! You may find that the muscles fatigue quickly at first, and that is OK! Your endurance can build with persistence! A marathon is not prepared for in one day. Many days of arduous training are needed to create a strong runner! Just like training for a long race, conditioning the pelvic floor muscles takes practice and rest. Practice and rest build strength. With strength comes control. With control comes continence in our own versions of a marathon, the marathon otherwise known as life…

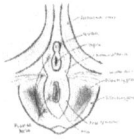

The Almighty Kegel!

Contracting the Pelvic Floor Muscles

Contracting or "squeezing" healthy pelvic floor muscles results in stopping the urine stream. This contraction of the pelvic floor muscles is known as a 'Kegel'. Kegels can also prevent defecation and engage during intercourse. The pelvic floor muscles, as depicted below, are aligned in a 'Figure 8' pattern. They act to close the orifices of the undersurface of the pelvic cavity.[1,2]

Here is an overview of the pelvic floor musculature:

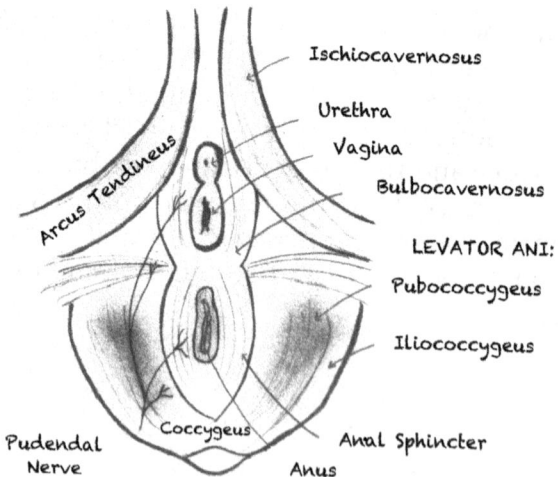

To introduce a Kegel, I often have a patient simulate an attempt to stop the urine flow. That is, in fact, what we are attempting to achieve in the realms of stress urinary incontinence and urinary urgency and frequency. I will often tell the patient to *test* the pelvic floor muscles once per week by commencing the urine stream, then stopping the flow midstream. With a successful Kegel, the patient can normally feel her/his pelvic floor muscles contract when the flow of urine slows or stops. This exercise can make use of the urine stream as a tactile cue and an audio cue, allowing the patient to feel and hear when (s)he finds the muscles that control urinary flow.

*Please note: I have always emphasized, and continue to emphasize, stopping the urine stream to test the pelvic floor's strength *only once per week* so as to not confuse the urinary system and create or enhance a problem with fully voiding.*

When performing in the clinic or practicing independently, I have the patient Kegel (contract the pelvic floor muscles) only as intensely and for as long as (s)he can in isolation of the stomach, buttocks, and inner thigh muscles (abdominals, gluteals, and adductors). Even if the intensity is minimal and even if the contraction or "squeeze" time is barely a second, isolation is key. Only with isolation achieved are the intensity and length of hold effective shields against incontinence.

When training a patient to isolate the pelvic floor, I have her/him place a hand on the muscles that are interfering with isolation, i.e., abdominals, gluteals, and adductors. This way, (s)he can feel when these accessory muscles are contracting and can attempt to disengage them. An alternative means to promote an isolated contraction of the pelvic floor is practicing the contraction while lying prone. If the abdominals contract, the patient may feel the abdomen lift up off the table, floor, or bed. Furthermore, in sitting, the patient may feel the altered seat pressure if (s)he contracts the gluteals. Performing a true Kegel can take some practice. However, these simple additions to the attempts can shorten the practice time needed to perform an isolated, and therefore effective, Kegel.

Isolation of the pelvic floor muscles is a difficult task for many patients. Contraction of the pelvic floor muscles may have been performed in conjunction with the contraction of other muscles for quite some time, and quite possibly without the knowledge of such. With concentration and cues, the patient can accomplish isolation. With proper training and practice, over time, the co-contraction habit can break, and a true Kegel can be achieved!

In most of my cases of pelvic floor muscle weakness, the patients have found it easiest to Kegel in supine, or lying down on her/his back. In supine, the contents of the pelvic cavity are not fully weighing on the pelvic floor or fully pressuring the orifices to open. In sitting, and even more so in standing, the contents' force on the pelvic floor can stretch apart the orifices like the mesh of a hammock that spreads when a person sits or lies on its threads. The lighter force in supine can make it easier for the pelvic floor muscles to close the orifices. Furthermore, in supine, the pelvic floor muscles do not have to work against gravity.

Side note: Standing on one's hands to Kegel would probably be the easiest of contraction attempts, but that task alone may pose a problem for some. Hanging upside down on a jungle gym or an inversion table may be better options to fully eliminate gravity. ;)

Learning to Kegel is only one segment of the road to recovery. Learning to time the Kegel *around* activities applies that newly found pelvic floor muscle strength to daily life! Kegeling around an activity means starting with a Kegel, performing an activity, then releasing the Kegel only after the activity has been completed. Kegeling makes the muscles strong, but it is the timing of that Kegel that can keep the leaks away while on the move!

Below are some tips on finding, strengthening, and timing the contraction of the pelvic floor muscles. Like training other muscles, Kegels should be performed in long durations for endurance, as quick repeats for agility training, and should be practiced around life's activities to make all that strengthening worthwhile!

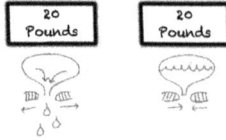

Pelvic Floor Exercises

Kegels: Pelvic floor muscle contractions or "squeezes".

- Once *(and only once)* per week, try to stop the flow of urine once you have started to void.
- While contracting the pelvic floor muscles, you should feel the pelvic floor being pulled toward your chest, drawn further into your body (upward if you are sitting or standing).
- Pillow trick:
  > Sitting on a soft pillow, contract the pelvic floor muscles so you can feel your undersurface, which is compressing the pillow, lift off the cushion.

Sustained Kegels: Long pelvic floor muscle contractions for endurance training.

- Contract the pelvic floor muscles (Kegel) for 10 seconds. Relax for 10-20 seconds.
- Repeat 10-second holds 10 times, 3-10 sets per day.

Quick Kegels: Quick contractions of the pelvic floor muscles for agility and for added bursts of strength.

- Contract the pelvic floor muscles (Kegel) as quickly as you can, contracting for only as long as is needed to feel a full squeeze, and only as firmly as you can in isolation. Preferable contractions are 2 seconds or less. Rest for 2-4 seconds between each contraction.
- Repeat 10 quick contractions 10 times, 3-10 sets per day.

Timing: Holding a Kegel *around* an activity. Start the Kegel *before* the activity, hold the Kegel *during* the activity, and release the Kegel *only after* the activity has been completed. Good times to practice are when standing from sitting, and when sitting from standing.

- Kegel, stand up, release the Kegel.
- Kegel, sit down, release the Kegel.
- Build your way up to holding the Kegel around multiple sit to stand exercises at once.

Timing exercises can help integrate Kegels into daily events that require the pelvic floor muscles to battle unwanted leakage. Such occurrences and activities include coughing, sneezing, and getting into and out of bed. The following are good times to practice!

- Kegel *around* a cough or sneeze:
    Kegel, cough or sneeze,
    release the Kegel.
- Kegel *around* getting into and out of bed:
    Kegel, get into or out of bed,
    release the Kegel.
- Gradually add activities around which to Kegel:
    Kegel *around* lifting an object or *around* stepping up and down a short flight of stairs.

Check, check, and check!

Endurance ☑

Agility ☑

Timing ☑

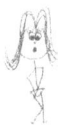

Combatting Urinary Urgency & Urinary Frequency

Kegels (pelvic floor muscle contractions) can suppress the urge to urinate by sending messages to the brain-bladder network to stop the bladder's contraction. In a successful situation, Kegeling signals the brain to turn off the bladder's detrusor muscle. Without the bladder's detrusor muscle contracting, the urine stops pressuring the internal sphincter to open. Without this pressure, the urge subsides and urine is retained until voiding is desired![34]

Kegels, or pelvic floor muscle contractions, (bottom right) send messages to the micturition center of the brain (upper left), which then signals the bladder (mid right) to stop contracting.[34]

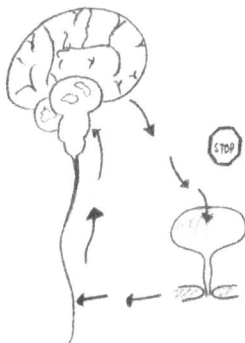

17

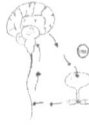

Suppressing an unwanted urge to urinate:

Pulsing quick Kegels can repeatedly message the brain to calm the bladder and keep it calm, thereby suppressing the urge to urinate.

1. If possible, sit down. If lying down when an urge strikes, remain in the lying position.
2. Perform 5-10 short bursts of Kegels, squeezing the pelvic floor muscles for only as long as you need to in order to feel a contraction, and only as firmly as you can in isolation.
3. Stay calm and determine if the urge to urinate has subsided.
4. If the urge has not been suppressed, repeat 5-10 short Kegels.
5. If lying down or sitting, hold a strong Kegel *around* the transfer to standing.
6. Calmly walk to the restroom while holding a moderate baseline Kegel and quickly pulsing stronger Kegels. This is similar to holding a rope, clenching your fist around the rope just enough so the rope does not drop, then clenching harder to resist someone pulling the rope out of your hand! If you are unable to release to the moderate hold without leaking, sustain a strong contraction while making your way to the restroom.
7. Void once the timing is appropriate.

1:00 PM   1:45 PM   2:30 PM

<u>Timed voiding</u>: Setting specific times to void throughout the day can catch the urgency before it strikes.

1. If urgency strikes once every hour, time your trip to the restroom every 45 minutes.
2. After the urgency is curbed, gradually increase the voiding intervals by 15 minutes. If sudden, uncontrollable urges resume, return to the more frequent voiding schedule.
3. The gradual increase in time between voids can help you gain control over the urge and eventually allow you to void in accordance with a full bladder.

Here is an example of a timed voiding schedule.

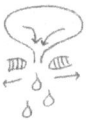

1:00 PM   1:45 PM   2:30 PM

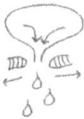

1:00 PM   2:00 PM   3:00 PM

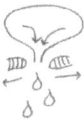

1:00 PM   2:15 PM   3:30 PM

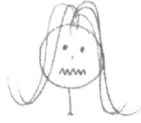

Pelvic Floor Muscle Pain & Incomplete Voiding

Excessive tension in the pelvic floor muscles can result from trauma and cause severe pain and difficulty urinating. Urinary urgency and frequency are often found in conjunction with incomplete voiding. A patient may stop the urine stream prematurely, or inadequately relax the pelvic floor muscles when trying to void. With residual urine in the bladder, the brain may think the bladder is still in *Go Mode*. Therefore, a few minutes later, the patient may need to rush back to the bathroom, often with extreme urgency, to void those last drops. Learning to relax the pelvic floor muscles with the *Lava Flow* exercise below can help fully relieve the bladder, and release painful tension!

Tension! = Pain! ➔ ➔ *Lava Flow ≈ Relief*

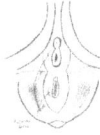

Releasing Pelvic Floor Muscle Tension

To relax the pelvic floor muscles: Kegel, then release in progressive waves as needed.

1. Kegel.
2. Release (un-Kegel) and gently exhale.
3. Exhale and release again.
4. Exhale and release a third time.

This exercise can be even more effective when performed while sitting on a large therapy ball. The contours of the ball fit nicely beneath the pelvic floor, allowing the patient to sense the pressure of the ball against the perineum. Progressive relaxation, while exhaling, will likely result in greater sensation of the ball against the perineum. The ball, therefore, acts as a tactile cue suggesting that relaxation is occurring. The sensation of tactile pressure on the perineum slowly moves *downward* with progressive relaxations. This exercise is easier to *feel* than to verbally describe. If you have access to a therapy ball, sit on it and release the pelvic floor muscles as stated. You will likely sense the pressure changes as your muscles relax. Given the conical shape that the ball assumes while the patient is sitting on it and the slow downward flow of tactile sensation, I have named this reverse Kegel exercise the *Lava Flow*. ☺

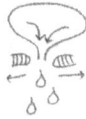

Helping the Bladder to Fully Empty

Difficulty emptying the bladder can be a nuisance and a time leach, as it is often accompanied by multiple trips to the restroom! Whether stemming from pelvic floor muscle tension, or dyssynergy among the bladder's contractions and the sphincters' openings, there are techniques aimed at easing the difficulty often experienced with urination. Combining the *Lava Flow* exercise with a few tricks listed below can improve urinary flow, freeing more time to spend outside of the restroom!

<u>**To assist with completely voiding**</u>: Apply the *Lava Flow* exercise to bathroom breaks!

- Blow[s] when you go! When voiding, blow[s] air through your mouth as if you are blowing through a flute. Concentrate on releasing the pelvic floor muscles with the *Lava Flow* technique as you blow.
- Stand up and sit down, then try voiding again. Once again, blow[s] when you go, and, think *Lava Flow*!
- Listen to running water, step into a warm shower, or think *Water Falls!* Blow[s] when you go, and think *Lava Flow*!

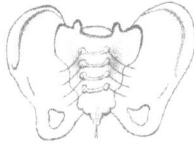

A Few Words Specifically for Men!

Learning to integrate long Kegels and quick, agility Kegels into daily activities, and learning to fully release the bladder contents with the *blow when you go* technique can help combat the effects of an enlarged prostate. For those opting for surgical removal of the prostate, a dose of *blowing when going* and learning to control the Kegel muscles *before* surgery can help dramatically before *and after* surgery! After surgery, sensing urinary leakage *and* sensing the whereabouts of the pelvic floor muscles can be difficult. Those two sensation deficiencies can add up to an incontinent disaster! Furthermore, pelvic floor muscle guarding after prostate surgery can wreak havoc on the ability to fully void. Incomplete voids, as stated previously, can lead to urinary urgency. Without the ability to find and hold the Kegel muscles, incontinence can thusly ensue. Patients who learn pelvic floor control techniques before surgery often find it much easier to gain or regain control of the pelvic floor post-operatively than those who do not. Take home messages? Learning how to Kegel and release can help combat prostate pressures, and if surgery is in the cards, learning to do so beforehand can make the road to recovery an easier one!

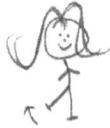

Your Very Own,
Personal Cheerleader

Strengthening the pelvic floor muscles with Kegels, timing those Kegels, and fully releasing the pelvic floor muscles can take practice! But, you can do it if you set your mind to it! Remember:

◆

Persist!

◆

Don't give up!

◆

Ye shall soon reap the benefits of your perseverance!

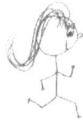

All My Best on
Your Kegel-ful Journey!

The above exercises aim to assist in gaining full control of the pelvic floor musculature. Whether the need be a stronger hold or an easier release, 'The Cheat Sheet' aims to help achieve the pelvic floor control needed to stay dry, minimize the number of needed bathroom breaks, and release harnessed tension!

I truly hope to have provided assistance with basic pelvic floor muscle control techniques. A multitude of confounding factors including disc herniations, neural impairments, prolapses, joint malalignments, and traumas can interfere with pelvic function. The information in 'The Cheat Sheet' just scratches the surface. But, it is a start! If you would like further information on rehabilitating pelvic dysfunction, including reducing pelvic pain associated with endometriosis and overcoming combined diagnoses, I recommend reading the full text version of 'Get the Pelvic Floor Back in Action'. I truly wish you a lifetime of fewer pelvic worries and more leak-free dances! Here's to running up mountains, instead of running to the restroom, and laughing 'til your belly aches, instead of laughing 'til your bladder bursts!! ☺

References

[1] Herschorn S MD, FRCSC. Female Pelvic Floor Anatomy: The Pelvic Floor, Supporting Structures, and Pelvic Organs. Rev Urol. 2004; 6(Suppl 5): S2–S10. Retrieved via http://www.ncbi.nlm.nih.gov/pmc/articles/PMC1472875/. August 23, 2014.

[2] Kegel AH MD, F.A.C.S. A Nonsurgical Method of Increasing the Tone of Sphincters and their Supporting Structures. 1948. Symposium presentation: Stress Incontinence and Genital Relaxation. CIBA Clinical Symposia, Feb-Mar 1952, Vol. 4, No. 2, pages 35-52. Retrieved via http://www.dothekegel.com/arnie/. August 23, 2014.

[3] http://www.hccfl.edu/media/383453/ch_25_summary.doc. Retrieved August 23, 2014.

[4] Fowler CJ, Griffiths D, de Groat WC. The Neural Control of Micturition. Nat Rev Neurosci. 2008 Jun; 9(6): 453–466. doi: 10.1038/nrn2401. Retrieved via http://www.ncbi.nlm.nih.gov/pmc/articles/PMC2897743/. October 1, 2014.

[5] Newman, D.K. (2002). New treatment options for overactive bladder and incontinence. The Director, 10(3).

Notes/Exercise Log